"Enhancing Stability

Quick and Easy 10-Minute Balance Workout for Seniors"

Miguel D. Solis),

Table of content

Introduction

Improving stability is a complex process that involves many different areas, from older citizens' personal well-being to international geopolitical issues. Fundamentally, it entails the adoption of policies and tactics meant to increase system equilibrium, reduce volatility, and promote resilience.

Developing coping strategies, building a sense of purpose, and strengthening mental and emotional resilience are some personal strategies for improving stability. It entails living a life that is consistently balanced, overcoming obstacles with flexibility, and laying the groundwork for long-term emotional health.

Stability in interpersonal relationships requires skillful communication, the capacity to resolve conflicts, and a dedication to mutual understanding. Creating strong relationships with others reinforces shared ideals and emotional stability in a supportive social setting.

Stability and adaptation are often associated at the organizational level. Establishing strong risk management procedures, fostering an innovative culture, and guaranteeing operational continuity are some of the ways that organizations and businesses try to improve stability. This strategy aids in an organization's capacity to withstand setbacks, preserve financial stability, and adjust to changing market circumstances.

Improving stability on a societal level entails tackling fundamental problems including political instability, social injustice, and economic inequality. A more stable and resilient society is achieved via enacting inclusive policies, encouraging social cohesiveness, and making investments in healthcare and education.

Increasing stability becomes a worldwide need in the international sphere. In order to promote global stability, diplomatic initiatives, dispute settlement, and cooperation on common problems like climate change and public health emergencies are essential. A more stable and secure international order is facilitated by multilateral collaboration and respect for international rules.

To sum up, the process of improving stability is a complex and multifaceted undertaking that involves aspects of the human, interpersonal, organizational, and social domains. We may have a positive impact on future generations and ourselves by taking proactive measures to solve obstacles, building resilience, and encouraging teamwork.

Important of stability

Global peace, social advancement, and individual well-being all depend on stability. Stability on a personal level offers a strong basis for mental and emotional well-being. It helps people overcome obstacles in life with fortitude, building confidence and a feeling of stability. Stable personal environments foster healthy connections, support the pursuit of long-term objectives, and enhance overall life happiness.

Stability is essential for building trust and cohesiveness in communities and relationships. Stability emphasizes predictability and dependability, two qualities that are essential to strong interpersonal relationships. Stability fosters peaceful relationships, clear communication, and a feeling of purpose among members of families, friendships, and broader social organizations.

Stability is a necessary component of economies and organizations for long-term development and success. When there is governmental stability, regulatory frameworks, and predictable market circumstances, businesses are able to flourish in a stable economic environment. Overall economic growth is facilitated by stability, which promotes investment, innovation, and the creation of employment opportunities.

Structural stability is fundamental to calm and forward-thinking societies on a larger scale. It entails dealing with problems like social injustice, poverty, and inequality in order to foster an atmosphere where people may thrive. Societies that are stable are better able to manage difficulties, encourage diversity, and provide opportunity to a wide range of people.

Global stability is essential for averting conflicts and promoting collaboration in the international sphere. A stable international order benefits nations by promoting diplomacy, cooperation in addressing global issues, and the peaceful settlement of conflicts. Global stability fosters cultural interaction, economic links, and the joint search for answers to common issues.

In conclusion, it is impossible to exaggerate the value of stability. It is the foundation that maintains social peace, personal fulfilment, and cross-border collaboration. We have a positive impact on a world where people can flourish, relationships can flourish, and long-term development can be maintained by actively appreciating and striving for stability.

Benefits of enhancing stability

Global peace, social advancement, and individual well-being all depend on stability. For most seniors, stability on a personal level offers a strong basis for mental and emotional well-being. It helps people overcome obstacles in life with fortitude, building confidence and a feeling of stability. Stable personal environments foster healthy connections, support the pursuit of long-term objectives, and enhance overall life happiness.

Stability is essential for building trust and cohesiveness in communities and relationships. Stability emphasizes predictability and dependability, two qualities that are essential to strong interpersonal relationships. Stability fosters peaceful relationships, clear communication, and a feeling of purpose among members of families, friendships, and broader social organizations.

Stability is a necessary component of economies and organizations for long-term development and success. When there is governmental stability, regulatory frameworks, and predictable market circumstances, businesses are able to flourish in a stable economic environment. Overall economic growth is facilitated by stability, which promotes investment, innovation, and the creation of employment opportunities.

Structural stability is fundamental to calm and forward-thinking societies on a larger scale. It entails dealing with problems like social injustice, poverty, and inequality in order to foster an atmosphere where people may thrive. Societies that are stable are better able to manage difficulties, encourage diversity, and provide opportunity to a wide range of people.

Global stability is essential for averting conflicts and promoting collaboration in the international sphere. A stable international order benefits nations by promoting diplomacy, cooperation in addressing global issues, and the peaceful settlement of conflicts. Global stability fosters cultural interaction, economic links, and the joint search for answers to common issues.

In conclusion, it is impossible to exaggerate the value of stability. It is the foundation that maintains social peace, personal fulfilment, and cross-border collaboration. We have a positive impact on a world where people can flourish, relationships can flourish, and long-term development can be maintained by actively appreciating and striving for stability.

Key element of stability

Stability in the human experience is a complex concept shaped by a multitude of interrelated factors. Emotional balance, or the capacity to weather life's ups and downs with fortitude, is one essential component. This stability is fostered by a high sense of self-awareness and emotional intelligence, which enables both young and elderly people to handle stress and keep their mental states stable.

Social stability, which entails fostering wholesome connections and a network of helpful people, is another essential component. A feeling of belonging, mental health, and stability in the face of adversity are all facilitated by human ties. These social underpinnings are constructed and maintained in large part via communication and trust.

Stability in one's career is crucial in the workplace. This calls for the acquisition and ongoing upgrading of skills, flexibility in the face of change, and a calculated approach to professional growth. In addition to being a major factor in general stability, a stable financial base enables people to confidently prepare for the future and satisfy their fundamental necessities.

Another essential component of stability is physical health. A healthy lifestyle that includes regular exercise, a well-balanced diet, and enough sleep promotes mental and physical toughness. Stability may be upset by health issues, emphasising the connection between physical and mental health.

Stability in education is essential for both individual development and society advancement. Intellectual stability is influenced by a person's access to high-quality education, ongoing learning, and capacity for change in response to changing information environments.

Human stability is also influenced by cultural and spiritual aspects, which provide people a sense of direction, morals, and a wider outlook. In order to navigate the difficulties of life, connecting with cultural customs and spiritual beliefs may provide direction, solace, and a moral compass.

The fundamental components of stability in the human form ultimately centre on a comprehensive strategy that takes into account aspects related to the emotional, social, professional, physical, educational, and cultural spheres. Through cultivating equilibrium and adaptability in all these aspects, people may effectively manage life's intricacies with an increased feeling of steadiness and welfare.

Factors affecting stability

During exercise, stability is affected by a number of variables, including:

Strength and Endurance of the Muscles: Stability is compromised by weak muscles, while stability is enhanced during movements by well-conditioned muscles that provide support and control.

Combined Adaptability: Sufficient range of motion in joints facilitates seamless and regulated motions, hence reducing the likelihood of instability.

Basis Strength: Stabilizing the spine and pelvis with a strong core provides a base for general stability in a variety of workouts.

Proprioception, or the body's awareness of where it is in space, and balance are essential for stability and depend on the nervous system, muscles, and sensory organs working together.

Surface and Footwear: Wearing the right shoes on level ground creates a strong foundation, which improves stability. Although unstable surfaces require balance and the activation of stabilizing muscles, they must be handled carefully.

Situation: In addition to ensuring ideal joint mechanics and minimizing the strain on muscles and ligaments, proper body alignment also adds stability to activity.

Equipment and Technique: Using the right workout equipment and using the right form are essential for stability. Inaccurate forms raise the possibility of instability and jeopardize joint integrity.

Age and Fitness Level: Aging-related changes in joint flexibility and muscle mass as well as general fitness level have an effect on stability. For people of all ages, regular exercise helps increase stability.

Control Neuromuscular: For coordinated motions to occur, the nervous system and muscles must communicate effectively. This has an impact on stability while doing dynamic workouts.

History of Injuries: Prior injuries may have an impact on muscle and joint function, necessitating focused therapy to rebuild strength and stop recurring instability.

Climatic Factors: During exercise, outside factors like temperature, light, and distractions may affect balance and attention.

Analytical Elements Stability is influenced by mental focus, attention, and confidence. A lack of focus or anxiety might affect stability and performance.

Diet and Hydration: Stability may be impacted by dehydration's effects on muscular function. Sufficient calorie intake is necessary for maintaining muscular function.

exhaustion and Recuperation: Muscle exhaustion brought on by overtraining and inadequate rest periods may undermine stability. Getting enough sleep is essential to continuing to function at your best.

Enhancing stability, lowering the risk of injuries, and increasing the general efficacy of exercise may all be attributed to knowing and taking care of these elements.

Warm up routine for age 50 above

Of course! The main goals of a well-rounded daily exercise programme for a 50-year-old should be to increase general mobility, strength, flexibility, and cardiovascular health. This is a potential strategy:

Comprehension (5–10 minutes): For the neck, shoulders, wrists, hips, knees, and ankles, begin with mild joint rotations.

For the purpose of raising heart rate and warming up the muscles, engage in mild aerobic exercise, such as marching in place or brisk jogging.

Exercise for the Heart (20–30 minutes): To strengthen your heart, take up exercises like cycling, swimming, dancing, running, or brisk walking.

Do your best to get in at least 150 minutes a week of aerobic activity at a moderate level.

Strength Training: two to three times a week Use resistance bands, small weights, or bodyweight movements to include resistance training.

Exercises for the main muscular groups should be included, such as planks and squats, lunges, push-ups, rows, and chest presses.

Adaptability and Speed (10–15 minutes): For every main muscle group, do dynamic stretches with an emphasis on increasing flexibility.

To improve range of motion overall, use static stretches and hold each pose for 15–30 seconds.

Stability and Balance (5–10 minutes):

Incorporate balance exercises including heel-to-toe walking, standing on one leg, and stability ball use.
Stability and balance may also be enhanced by practicing yoga or tai chi.

Core Exercises: Ten minutes, two to three times a week

Incorporate core-focused workouts like Russian twists, planks, and crunches.

In addition to promoting general stability, a strong core helps stave against lower back problems.

Relax and stretch for five to ten minutes]: Cool down in the end to gradually reduce heart rate.

To increase flexibility and decrease muscular tension, do static stretches for your main muscle groups.

Optional Mind-Body Exercise: To support mental health and reduce stress, think about engaging in yoga or meditation.

Rehydration and Hydration: Drink enough water before, during, and after working out.

Ample rest and recuperation time should be allotted in between sessions.

Before beginning a new fitness regimen, always get medical advice, particularly if you have any pre-existing medical concerns. Based on your own fitness level, modify the length and intensity of your workouts and make steady development over time.

Seated exercises

Exercises that are done while seated provide a flexible and easily accessible means of adding movement to one's routine. These exercises are beneficial for those who have limited mobility, are recuperating from injuries, or are just searching for low-impact training choices. This is a thorough examination of sitting workouts for many fitness domains:

Sitting Cardiovascular Exercises:

sitting Marching: Using your core muscles, raise and drop your knees in a marching motion while sitting.

Seated Jumping Jacks: Replicate the classic jumping jack action by simultaneously extending your arms and legs outward.

Cyclist Crunches While Seated: Sit up straight and raise your legs to your chest alternatively, simulating a riding action.

Sitting Strength Training Exercises:

Lunges with the Seat: Using the leg muscles, straighten one or both legs and raise them off the ground.

Recreation in Seats: To target the back muscles while sitting, mimic a rowing action using resistance bands or light weights.

Seated Dumbbell push: Using your arms and shoulders, push the dumbbells above while maintaining shoulder height.

Exercises for Flexibility and Mobility While Seated:

Seated Forward Bend: Stretch your lower back and hamstrings by sitting with your legs outstretched and reaching forward to your toes.

Seated Torso rotate: To increase spinal flexibility, sit up straight and rotate your upper body to one side, then the other.

Seated Neck Stretches: To release tension and encourage neck flexibility, gently tilt your head forward and to either side.

Balance and Stability Activities While Seated:

sitting Leg Crosses: While sitting, cross one leg over the other, using your core muscles to maintain balance.

Seated Heel Taps: Test your stability by lifting one heel at a time while maintaining the rest of your foot on the ground.

Seated Knee Extensions: To improve stability, extend one leg at a time while momentarily keeping it in place.

Meditation on the Mind-Body Connection:

Seated Meditation: To encourage calmness and mental health, sit down and practise mindfulness and deep breathing.

Seated Yoga postures: Modify standing postures to sit-only variations, emphasising breathing and soft motions.

sitting Tai Chi exercises: To enhance balance and concentration, use contemplative and flowing Tai Chi exercises while sitting.

Seated Interval Exercises:
Seated High Knees: For quick bursts of high-intensity exercise, raise your knees quickly in a marching motion.

Arm Circles in Seats: For interval training, rotate your arms in little or big circles while progressively increasing your pace.

Chair-Based Resistance Exercises for Sitting:

sitting Chest Press: To simulate a chest press while sitting, use dumbbells or resistance bands.

Seated Bicep Curls: Work your arm muscles by doing bicep curls with weights or resistance bands.

Routine for Seated Stretching:

Sitting Side Extend: To stretch your obliques, extend one arm overhead and slant to the side.

Hips flexor stretch in a sitting: To stretch the hip flexors, cross one ankle over the other knee and apply little pressure.

Shoulder Stretch in Sitting: Extend your shoulders by bringing one arm across your chest and applying little pressure to the upper arm.

A well-rounded approach to fitness may be achieved by include a number of sitting exercises in a regimen, which can accommodate a range of fitness levels and objectives. Before beginning a new fitness regimen, always get advice from a medical practitioner or fitness specialist, particularly if you have any underlying medical issues.

Standing Poses

A fundamental component of many workout regimens, standing poses enhance strength, balance, flexibility, and general health. Standing postures provide a variety of advantages whether they are used in yoga, strength training, or daily mobility. This is a thorough investigation of standing positions in many fitness domains.

Standing Poses for Yoga:

Mountain Pose (Tadasana): Raise your arms aloft, ground through your feet, and stand tall with your feet together.

Warrior I (Virabhadrasana I): Engage the whole body by stepping one foot back, bending the front knee, and extending the arms aloft.

Tree Pose (Vrksasana): Reach your arms upwards while maintaining balance on one leg and placing the sole of your other foot on your inner thigh or calf.

Standing Poses for Strength Training:

Squats: While keeping your feet shoulder-width apart, squat down, using your thighs and glutes to propel yourself forward.

Longines: Work your lower body by putting one foot forward, bending both knees, and lowering the rear knee towards the floor.

Raises the Calf: To strengthen your calf muscles, stand up on the balls of your feet.

Stability and Balance Standing Positions: Single Leg Balance: Raising one foot off the floor, use your core and stabilising muscles to balance on the other.
Heel-to-Toe Walk: To improve balance, walk in a straight line while putting one foot's heel in front of the other's toes.

Tuladandasana, or Balancing Stick Pose: Lean forward and extend one leg straight back, reaching forward with the arms for balance.

Standing Positions for Flexibility and Mobility:

Forward Fold (Uttanasana): Extend your lower back and hamstrings by extending your hips and reaching towards the floor.

Standing Side Stretch: Lean to the side and extend one arm above to stretch the body's side.

Quad Stretch: To stretch the quadriceps, bend one knee and bring the foot up to the glutes.

Standing Pose for Mind-Body Connection: Mountain Pose with Mindful Breathing: Take a tall stance, concentrate on your breathing, and pay attention to every breath you take in and out.

Standing Meditation: While standing, firmly plant your feet, shut your eyes, and engage in mindful awareness exercises.

Mindful Walking: Move slowly and deliberately while focusing on each stride and feeling.

Standing Positions for Functional Movement: Functional Squats: these exercises emphasize good form for daily functioning by simulating sitting and standing actions.

Standing Leg Swings: To increase hip mobility, swing one leg forth and backward.

Lift one leg to the side while using your outer hip muscles to do side leg raises.
Compact Training with Standing Positions:

Jumping Jacks: Combine cardio into standing postures by jumping with your feet apart and your arms raised over your head. Then, leap back to your starting position.

Knees up: For quick bursts of high-intensity aerobics, quickly lift your knees towards your chest.

Box Leaps: Elevate your strength and agility by either stepping onto a firm platform or engaging in pretend box jumps.

Positions for Postural Alignment Standing:

Posture Check: Place your back against a wall and make sure your head, shoulders and hips are in the right positions.
Tadasana with Shoulder Blade Retraction: To improve posture, stand tall and engage your shoulder blades.

Standing poses are a great way to target different parts of physical fitness and provide variety to your workout programme. Always use good form while practicing, and if you have any particular health issues or diseases, you should think about getting advice from a fitness specialist.

Prop-Based Stability Drills

By adding props to stability exercises, you may make your exercise regimen more dynamic and demanding while improving your balance, strength, and flexibility. This is a thorough examination of many muscle groups and general stability-enhancing prop-based stability drills:

Bosu Ball Workouts:

Bosu Ball Squats: To work your core and lower body, stand on the flat side of the Bosu ball and execute squats.

Lunges with a bosom: Put one foot on the Bosu ball and do forward or lateral lunges to test your leg muscles and stability.

Drills using Stability Balls:

Planks with Stability Balls: Using the shoulder and core stabilizers, place your hands on a stability ball and assume a plank posture.

Stability Ball Hamstring Curls: To work your glutes and hamstrings, move the stability ball towards you while lying on your back with your feet on it.

Exercises using Balance Discs:

Disc with Single-Leg Balance: Using a balancing disc, stand on one leg to test your ankle proprioception and stability.

Balance Disc Squats: To exercise your lower body more, squat with one or both feet on a balancing disc.

How Resistance Band Stability Works

Y-Walks with Resistance Bands: To strengthen your ankles and target your hip abductors, wrap a resistance band over them and go on lateral walks.

Resistance Band Rotational Exercises: To work your core muscles, secure a resistance band to a fixed place and rotate.

Exercises for TRX Suspension Trainers:

TRX Handgun Lunges: To emphasize leg strength and balance, execute pistol squats with the help of TRX straps.

Training for Single-Leg Lunges: Do lunges with one foot hanging in TRX straps to test your stability.

Medicine Ball Exercises for Stability:

Single-leg Romanian deadlifts using medicine balls: To improve balance and work the posterior chain, do single-leg RDLs while holding a medicine ball.

Medicine Ball Wood Chops: Use a medicine ball to do woodchop movements that will activate your core muscles.

Training for Foam Roller Stability:

Foam Roller Plank: To test stability and activate core muscles, place your hands on a foam roller and assume a plank posture.

One-Leg Foam Roller Bridge: To work on your glutes and hamstrings, elevate one foot on a foam roller and execute bridges.

Ankle Weights for Stability in the Lower Body:

Ankle Weight Leg Lifts: To work the muscles in your outer thighs and hip flexors, put on ankle weights and execute leg lifts.

Knee Extensions with Ankle Weight: To engage your quadriceps, sit on a stability ball and execute knee extensions while wearing ankle weights.

Drills for Kettlebell Stability:

Kettlebell Deadlifts with Just One Leg:
Use a kettlebell to do one-leg deadlifts to strengthen your posterior chain and improve your balance.

Kettlebell Windmills: This exercise tests your stability by focusing on your shoulder and core stabilizers.

Strengthening using Dumbbells:

Dumbbell Step-Ups on an unsteady Surface: To work your lower body muscles, step up onto an unsteady surface while carrying dumbbells.

One-leg dumbbell overhead press Use dumbbells to execute overhead lifts while standing on one leg to test your balance and shoulder stability.

Drills for Agility Ladders: On the Agility Ladder, the Lateral ShuffleOn an agility ladder, do lateral shuffles to develop your footwork and lateral stability.

High Knees Through Ladder: By practicing high knees through an agility ladder, you may raise your heart rate and improve your balance.

Exercises for Pilates Ring Stability:

Ring Squeezes in Pilates: Squeeze the Pilates ring between your thighs to strengthen your inner thighs and improve your stability.

Pilates Ring Plank with Knee Tucks: Squeeze a Pilates ring and do knee tucks to intensify a plank posture.

Cone Drilling for Stability in Motion:

Hop cones: Arrange cones and quickly jump from side to side to work your lower body muscles and enhance your dynamic stability.

Zig-Zag Cone Jumps: To test your agility and lower body stability, jump around cones in a zigzag fashion.

Work on Stability using Yoga Blocks: Yoga Block Balancing: To improve ankle stability, practice balancing on one leg while standing on a yoga block.

Yoga Block Squats: To increase resistance and test your stability, squat while holding a yoga block.

Stability Circuit Based on Props:

Make a Circuit: For a thorough workout, include a variety of prop-based stability exercises into a circuit.

Rotate between several prop-based exercises as you go through each exercise to target different muscle groups and enhance your overall stability.

These prop-based stability exercises can help you successfully test and improve your balance while working out a variety of muscle groups in your training regimen. Always use correct form, begin at a manageable difficulty level, then increase progressively as your stability increases. Personalized advice based on your fitness level and objectives may be obtained by consulting with a fitness specialist.

Daily Activities to Improved Stability in general

Including regular exercises aimed at improving stability is a good approach to enhance general health and lower the chance of injury. These exercises, which range from easy motions to deliberate ones, help to increase flexibility, strength, and balance. Now let's investigate everyday activities in more detail for improved stability:

Morning Stretching Routine: Stretching gently first thing in the morning helps to awaken the muscles and joints.

For the purpose of increasing flexibility and mobility, use exercises like contacting toes, reaching upwards, and mild twisting.

One-Leg Balancing: To improve your balance, try standing on one leg while waiting in line or brushing your teeth.

Slowly extend the time and difficulty by shutting your eyes or adding little motions.

Practical Workouts for Cooking: Leg rises and side leg raises may be stabilised by using the kitchen counter.

While you wait for the water to boil, do squats or calf raises. Make strength training a part of your everyday routine.

Tranquil Walking: Be mindful of your gait and make sure you're moving from heel to toe correctly.

Walking with intention and paying attention to every stride enhances stability and fosters awareness.

Climbing Stairs: When feasible, use the stairs, with special focus on good balance and coordination.

As your stability increases, progressively increase the intensity while holding onto the railing for support.

Workplace Seat Exercises: To keep your circulation and flexibility up, do sitting leg lifts, ankle circles, and seated torso twists at your desk.

March while sitting to strengthen your core and increase blood flow.

Strolling over uneven terrain: Incorporate strolls on grass, pebbles, or uneven ground to test your stability.

Be mindful of your footing and contract your ankle, knee, and hip stabilizing muscles.

At-Home Functional Movements: When doing domestic tasks or picking up goods, use motions like squatting.

To strengthen your lower body, practise standing up from a sitting posture without using your hands.

Tai Chi or Yoga Breaks: Throughout the day, take brief pauses to do basic Tai Chi or yoga stretches.

The focus of these workouts is on balance, flexibility, and deliberate movement.

Conscious Seating: When sitting, concentrate on keeping your back straight and your weight properly distributed across both hips.

To strengthen your general stability and support your spine, use your core muscles. **Activities using a Balance Board or Stability Ball:**For an extra challenge, include a stability ball or balancing board into your practice.

Standing on these unsteady surfaces, do workouts like squats or light motions.

Activities Outside: Take part in outdoor pursuits including nature hikes, hiking, and trail walking.

The possibility to challenge and enhance stability is greatly enhanced by the varied terrain and natural components.

Yard or Gardening Work:

Planting and weeding are two examples of gardening tasks that need a variety of actions that improve stability.

During these activities, pay attention to appropriate weight distribution and body mechanics.

Spinning: Whether it's in a formal classroom setting or during unscheduled dancing breaks at home, include dance into your daily routine.

Coordination, rhythm, and general body awareness are all enhanced by dancing.

Activities in the Water:A low-impact method of building muscle and improving stability is swimming or water aerobics.

Water's buoyancy acts as resistance without straining joints.

You may gradually increase your stability, lower your chance of falling, and improve your general physical well-being by including these everyday exercises into your routine. When engaging in these exercises, consistency and attention are essential for achieving the long-term advantages of increased stability. Always pay attention to your body's signals, and if you have any particular health issues, get advice from a medical practitioner or fitness specialist.

Monitoring Balance Improvement

It's critical to monitor and measure balance development in order to evaluate progress, pinpoint problem areas, and guarantee a safe and successful fitness journey. Here is a thorough examination of techniques and factors to take into account while tracking balance improvement:

Initial Evaluation: Start by evaluating your present balancing skills on a baseline basis.

To assess initial stability, use basic tasks like standing on one leg while closing and opening your eyes.

Keeping Documents:
MKeep a notebook or use a fitness app to log your observations, routines, and balancing exercises.
Keep track of any stability shifts, difficulties encountered, and advancements over time.

Evaluations of Balance: Review balance evaluations on a regular basis to evaluate progress objectively.

To evaluate certain facets of stability, use standardized balancing tests or consult with a fitness specialist.

Tests of Functional Movement: Include functional mobility assessments that replicate real-world situations, including getting up from a sitting posture or walking over uneven terrain.

Analyzing balance in real-world situations provides light on daily stability.

Challenges Based on Time: As stability improves, progressively increase the length of balancing exercises by setting specific time-based challenges.

For instance, try maintaining a one-legged stance for a prolonged amount of time, increasing the challenge over many weeks or months.

Utilizing Wearable Technology

Think of using wearable technology that monitors balance and movement.

There are fitness trackers and smartwatches that measure parameters relating to balance, steps, and gait.

Analysis of the Video: Make videos of yourself doing balancing exercises so you can review your technique and see where you need to improve.

Examine films side by side over time to see how posture, stability, and movement patterns develop.

Comments from peers or trainers: Ask for advice from physical therapists, fitness instructors, or exercise partners.

External observations might provide insightful information about areas that can benefit from change or attention.

Subjective Self-Evaluation: Evaluate your feelings both during and after balancing workouts on a regular basis.

Note any changes in your sense of general movement confidence, muscular engagement, or perceived stability.

Exercises for Functional Balance: Include functional balancing exercises in your everyday routines and activities.

Practice waiting in line while standing on one leg, for instance, or add balancing exercises to your strength training routine.

Incremental Difficulty: To keep pushing yourself, go gradually through the balancing exercises' increasing levels of difficulty.

This can include introducing dynamic motions, broadening the range of motion, or creating instability.

Recurrent Evaluation: Plan frequent evaluation periods to monitor long-term development.

To measure progress over longer time periods, review baseline evaluations and compare outcomes.

Being Aware of the Environment: Keep in mind that external elements like uneven surfaces or changing lighting might affect equilibrium.

Adapt your programme in light of these considerations to keep your balance training environment safe and productive

Paying Attention to Your Body: Observe your body's reaction to various balancing exercises.

Identify symptoms of exhaustion, tense muscles, and any pain that would suggest adjustments are necessary.

Combining with Overall Fitness Objectives: Sync up balance monitoring with more general fitness objectives.

For instance, concentrate on balancing exercises that are appropriate for your particular sport or activity if your objective is to improve athletic performance.

You can efficiently evaluate and enhance stability over time by combining objective evaluations, subjective observations, and ongoing changes to your balancing practice. A comprehensive and long-lasting path to balance development involves regular self-reflection and a holistic approach to training. Always seek advice from medical professionals or fitness specialists, particularly if you have any pre-existing health issues or concerns.

Setting Realistic Goals

Whether in terms of one's personal, professional, or physical growth, setting reasonable objectives is essential. Setting and achieving realistic objectives offers direction, inspiration, and a feeling of success. Here is a thorough examination of the guidelines and factors to take into account while creating realistic goals:

Introspection: Start by taking stock of your present skills, resources, and obligations.

Think about the time and effort you can realistically commit to achieving your objectives, as well as your strengths and shortcomings.

SMART-T Requirements: Make your objectives precise, quantifiable, attainable, relevant, and time-bound by using the S.M.A.R.T. criterion.

Your objectives will be easier to achieve thanks to this framework's assurance of clarity and viability.

Long-Term vs. Short-Term Objectives:

Differentiate between your long-term and short-term objectives.

Short-term goals make development more achievable and quantifiable by serving as stepping stones towards long-term objectives.

Dissect Bigger Objectives: Segment more ambitious objectives into more manageable phases.

This strategy avoids feeling overwhelmed and instead encourages a feeling of accomplishment with every milestone.

Take Resources and Constraints into Account: Evaluate possible limitations, like time, money, or other obligations.

Realistic objectives are more doable since they match the resources at hand.

Highest Priorities: Set priorities for your goals according to their importance, urgency, or compatibility with your larger life goals.

It is more clear and committed to focus on a small number of important objectives at a time.

Take Failures Into Account: Recognise that obstacles are an inevitable element of every endeavor.

Be reasonable in your expectations by acknowledging that growth isn't always straight forward.

Freedom and Adaptability: Remain flexible in the face of shifting conditions.

Goals should be adjusted as necessary, particularly if new facts or unforeseen occurrences occur.

Incorporate Gradual Adjustments: Make small adjustments at first to prevent overstretching yourself.

Gradual development fosters confidence and creates enduring habits.

Conform to Personal Principles: Make sure your objectives are in line with your dreams and basic principles.

A stronger feeling of purpose arises when you pursue objectives that align with your beliefs.

Recognise Little Victories: Celebrate and give thanks for little victories along the road.

Acknowledging accomplishments encourages drive and a good outlook.

Create a Support Network: Tell your network of supporters what your aims are.

Possessing responsibility and encouragement boosts the chances of achievement.

Timely Evaluation and Modification: Review your objectives and your progress on a regular basis.

If required, modify schedules or tactics to maintain consistency with your changing priorities

Setting Mindful Objectives: Make sure your ambitions are driven by internal desire rather than by outside pressure.

Objectives motivated by a person's interest and passion are more likely to be accomplished.

Ask for expert advice: Think about consulting experts for help in areas such as career guidance or fitness.

A systematic strategy and reasonable expectations are provided by expert assistance.

Keep Ambition and Realism in Check: Strike a balance between having big dreams and being grounded in reality.

Growth is fueled by ambition, but ambition has to be balanced with an awareness of your existing limitations.

Assess and Understand: Analyze your development on a regular basis and take lessons from your mistakes.

Recognise what worked successfully and what changes might improve your strategy moving forward.

Aim in Harmony with Lifestyle: Make sure your objectives complement your general way of life and wellbeing.

Sustainability is encouraged when you pursue objectives that enhance your lifestyle rather than cause conflict.
A Positive Attitude: By concentrating on what you can control and praising your accomplishments, you may foster a positive mentality.
Persistence and resilience are aided by optimism.

Grasp the Adventure: Realize that the process of achieving a goal is just as important as the final destination.

Accepting the process increases one's feeling of fulfillment in general.

A dynamic and individualized process, setting realistic objectives calls for careful thinking, self-awareness, and a dedication to ongoing progress. You may build an approachable and personally relevant framework for success by integrating these ideas into your goal-setting process.

Conclusion

In summary, stability is a critical investment that seniors and general people should make in order to preserve their autonomy and general well-being as they age. Stability improvement via a multimodal approach that includes strength, flexibility, balance, and cognitive components becomes more and more important in order to provide a strong and stable base.

As we age, a customized fitness programme must take into account and address characteristics like muscular strength, joint flexibility, and balance. Incorporating exercises such as weight training, balancing routines, and flexibility routines may greatly improve stability, lower the chance of falling, and boost self-assurance while doing everyday tasks.

Furthermore, it's critical to acknowledge the uniqueness of every senior's health situation and modify exercise regimens appropriately. A comprehensive approach to well-being and regular check-ins with medical specialists may help elders embark on a customized and sustained stability improvement path.

In this endeavor, encouraging an optimistic outlook and acknowledging accomplishments of any size enable elders to choose a more stable and active lifestyle. Seniors may enjoy their golden years with confidence and vigor as a result of these efforts, which not only improve the body but also foster a feeling of self-efficacy, resilience, and independence.